In a world inundated with fad diets, quick fixes, and unrealistic expectations, the journey to weight loss can often feel overwhelming and daunting. Yet, at its core, weight loss is not just about shedding pounds; it's a profound journey of self-discovery, empowerment, and transformation.
Welcome to "A Holistic Approach to Weight Loss: 82 Chapters of Transformation." In this comprehensive guide, we delve deep into the multifaceted aspects of weight loss, offering insights, strategies, and inspiration

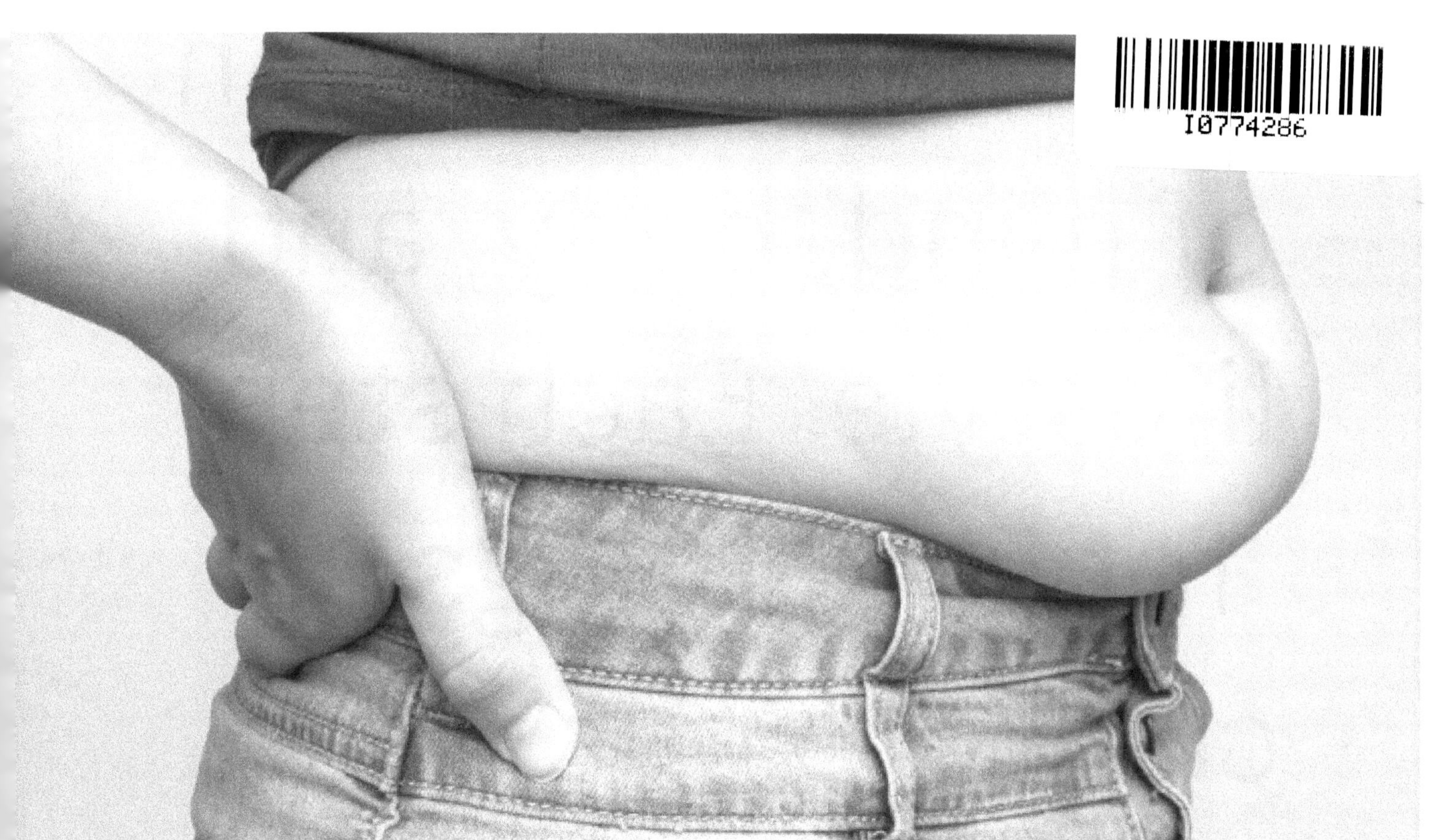

Chapter 1: Introduction

Embarking on a weight loss journey is more than just shedding pounds; it's a transformation of mind, body, and lifestyle. Each step forward brings us closer to our goals.

Chapter 2: Setting Goals

Setting clear, achievable goals is crucial in any weight loss journey. Whether it's fitting into a favorite dress or improving overall health, defining what you want to achieve is the first step

Chapter 3: Understanding Nutrition

Nutrition is the cornerstone of weight loss. Learning about macronutrients, portion sizes, and balanced meals empowers us to make healthier choices and fuel our bodies effectively.

Chapter 4: The Role of Exercise

Exercise not only burns calories but also strengthens muscles and improves cardiovascular health. Finding activities we enjoy makes staying active a sustainable part of our routine

Chapter 5: Overcoming Obstacles

Challenges are inevitable on the path to weight loss. By identifying potential obstacles and developing strategies to overcome them, we can stay resilient and focused on our goals

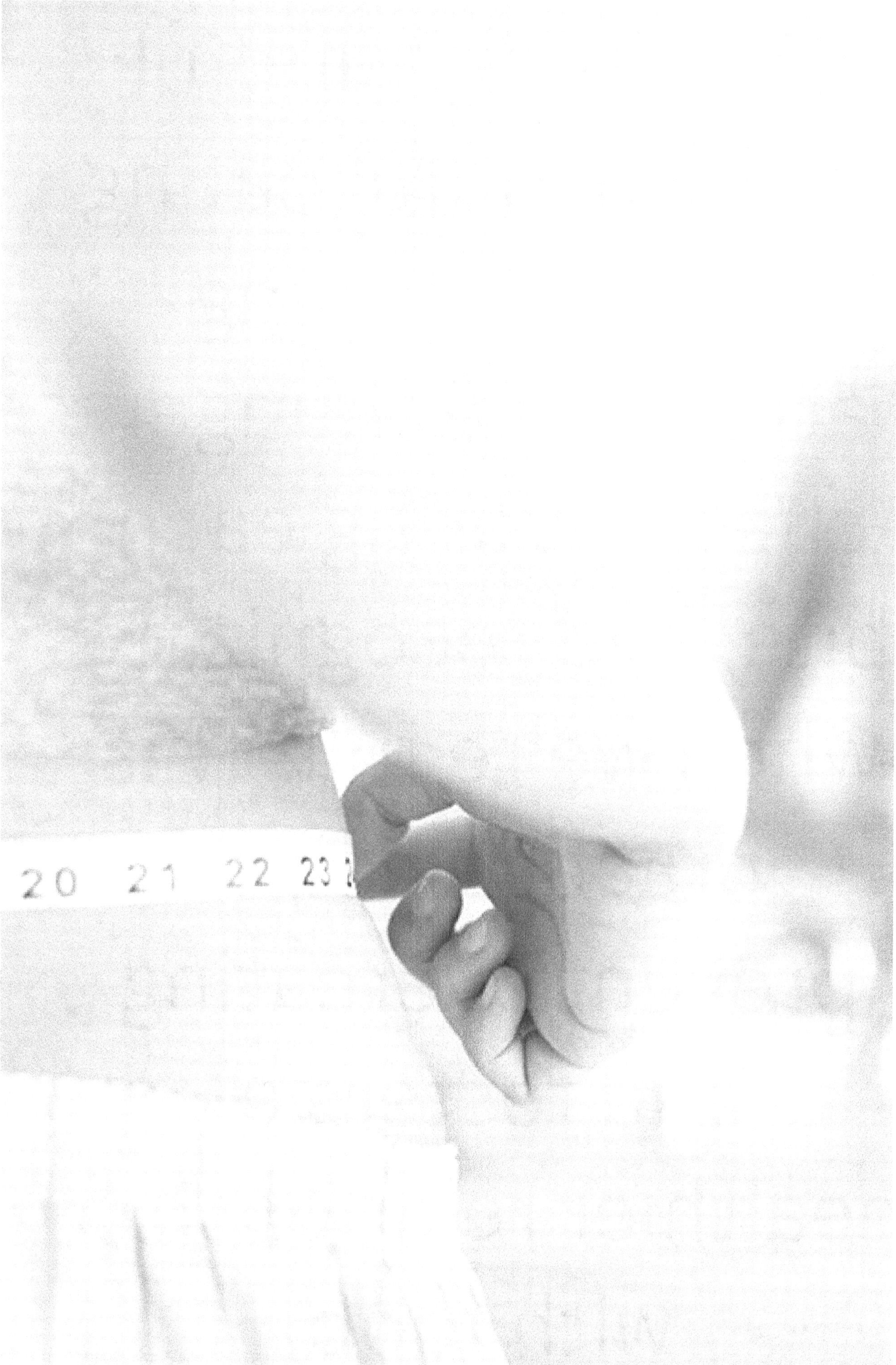

20 21 22 23

Chapter 6: Mindful Eating

Mindful eating involves paying attention to hunger cues, savoring each bite, and recognizing when we're full. This practice helps prevent overeating and fosters a healthier relationship with foob

Chapter 7: Building Healthy Habits

Consistency is key in weight loss. By gradually incorporating healthy habits into our daily lives, we create a sustainable foundation for long-term success

Chapter 8: Tracking Progress

Monitoring progress through measurements, photos, or journaling provides valuable feedback and motivation. Celebrating milestones, no matter how small, keeps us inspired to continue

Chapter 9: Managing Stress

Stress can sabotage weight loss efforts by triggering emotional eating and disrupting sleep patterns. Incorporating stress-reduction techniques such as meditation or yoga promotes overall well-being.

Chapter 10: Getting Quality Sleep

Adequate sleep is essential for weight loss and overall health. Prioritizing sleep hygiene habits, such as a consistent bedtime routine and creating a restful sleep environment, improves both the quantity and quality of sleep

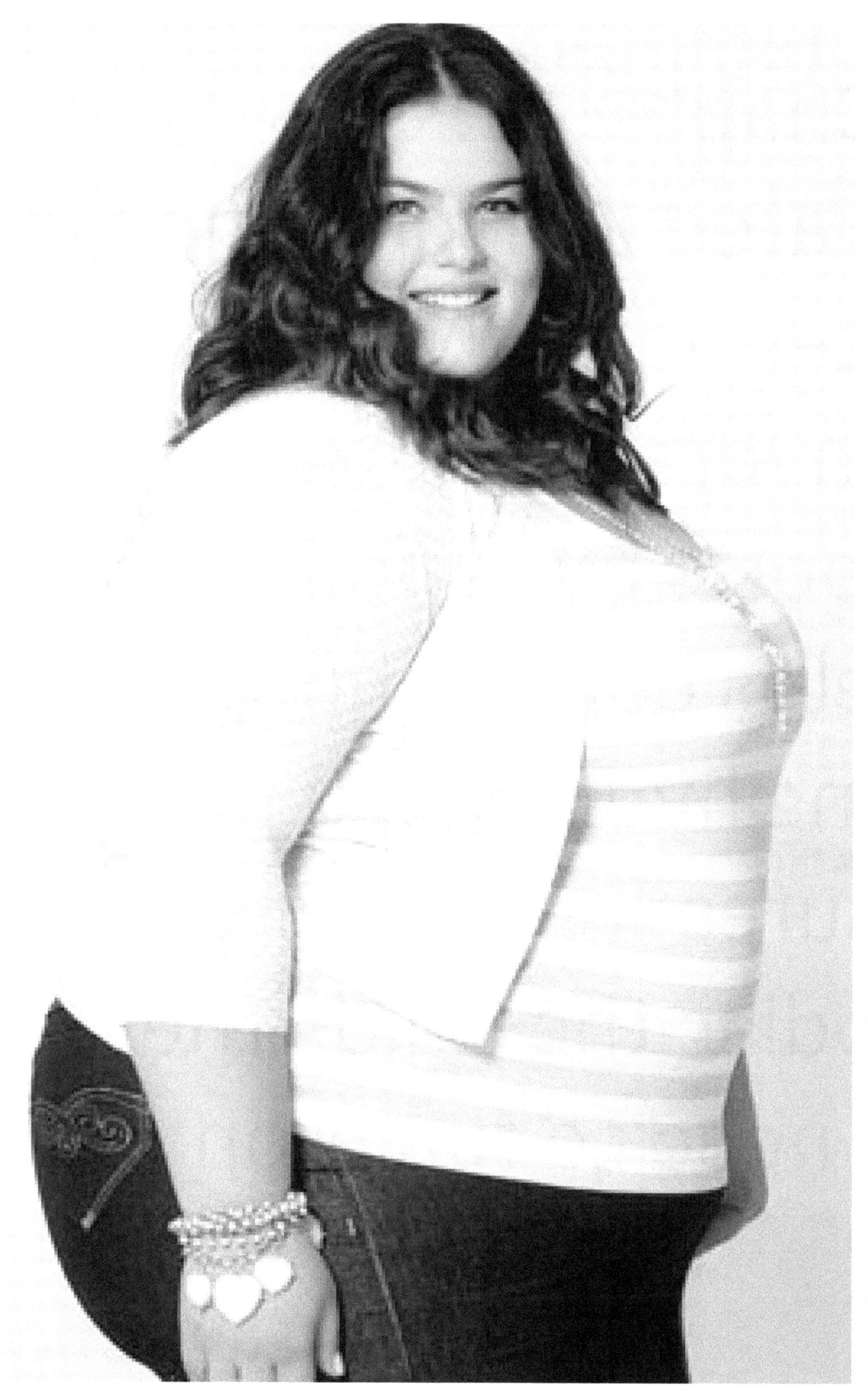

Chapter 11: Staying Hydrated

Drinking enough water not only keeps us hydrated but also supports metabolism and helps control hunger. Making hydration a priority ensures we're giving our bodies the fluids they need to function optimally.

Surrounding ourselves with a supportive community can make all the difference in our weight loss journey. Whether it's friends, family, or online groups, having people who understand and encourage us can keep us motivated

Chapter 13: Creating a Meal Plan

Meal planning saves time, money, and stress while promoting healthier eating habits. By preparing meals ahead of time and having nutritious options readily available, we're less likely to make impulsive food choices.

Chapter 14: Incorporating Variety

Variety is the spice of life – and the key to preventing boredom in our diet. Experimenting with new recipes, cuisines, and ingredients keeps healthy eating exciting and enjoyable

Chapter 15: Dealing with Plateaus

Plateaus are a natural part of any weight loss journey. Instead of getting discouraged, we can use plateaus as an opportunity to reassess our habits, make adjustments, and reignite progres

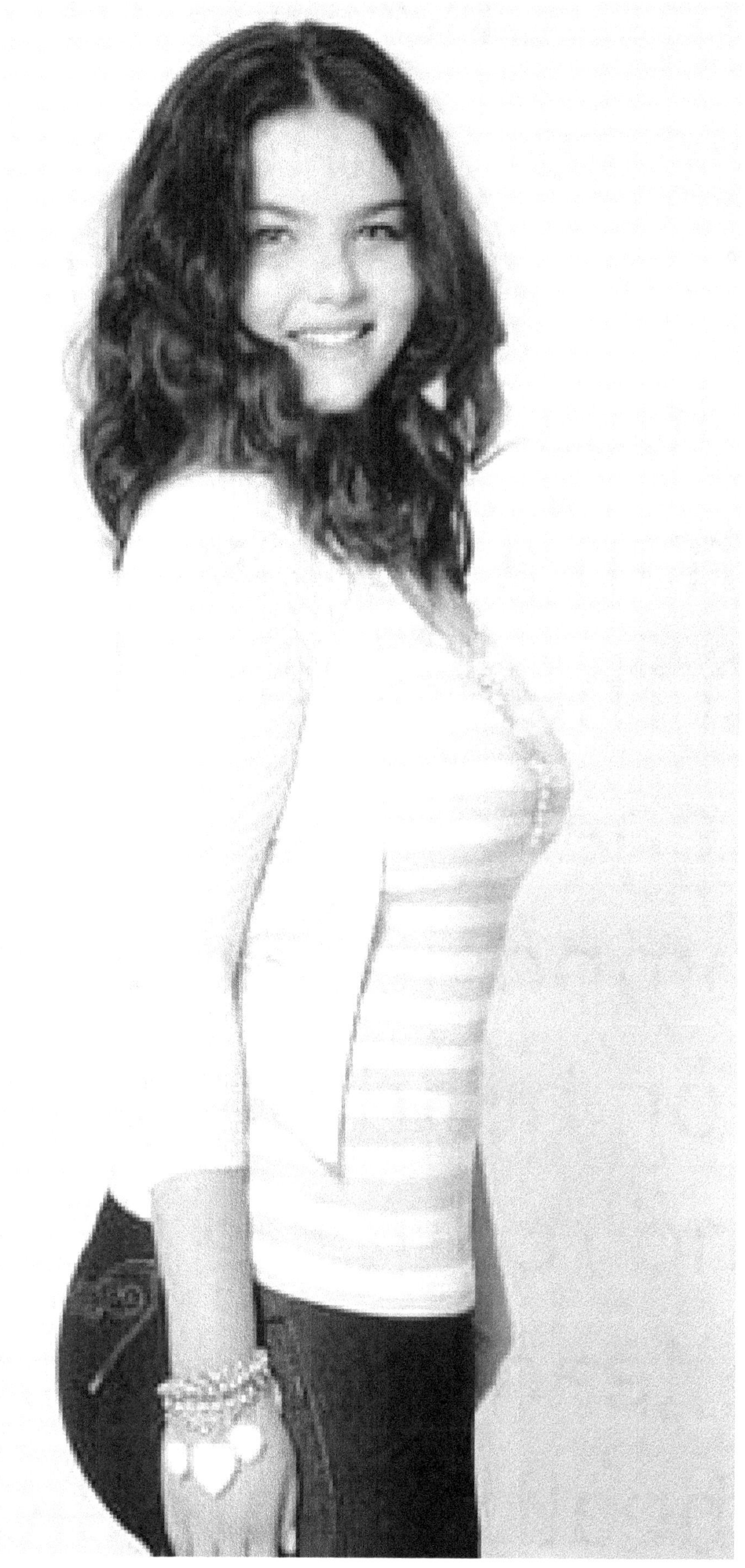

Chapter 16: Understanding Body Composition

Weight loss is about more than just the number on the scale; it's about changing our body composition. Focusing on building muscle and reducing body fat leads to a leaner, healthier physique.

Chapter 17: Embracing Imperfection

Perfection is unattainable – and unnecessary – in our weight loss journey. Embracing imperfection allows us to learn from setbacks, adapt, and continue moving forward with compassion and resilience

Chapter 18: Seeking Professional

Guidance Consulting with healthcare professionals, such as registered dietitians or personal trainers, provides personalized guidance and support tailored to our individual needs and goals

Chapter 19: Creating a Supportive Environment

Our physical surroundings play a significant role in shaping our behaviors and habits. By creating asupportive environment that promotes healthy choices, we set ourselves up for success

Chapter 20: Overcoming Emotional Eating

Emotional eating is a common challenge in weight loss. Developing alternative coping strategies, such as journaling or engaging in hobbies, helps us address underlying emotions without turning to food.

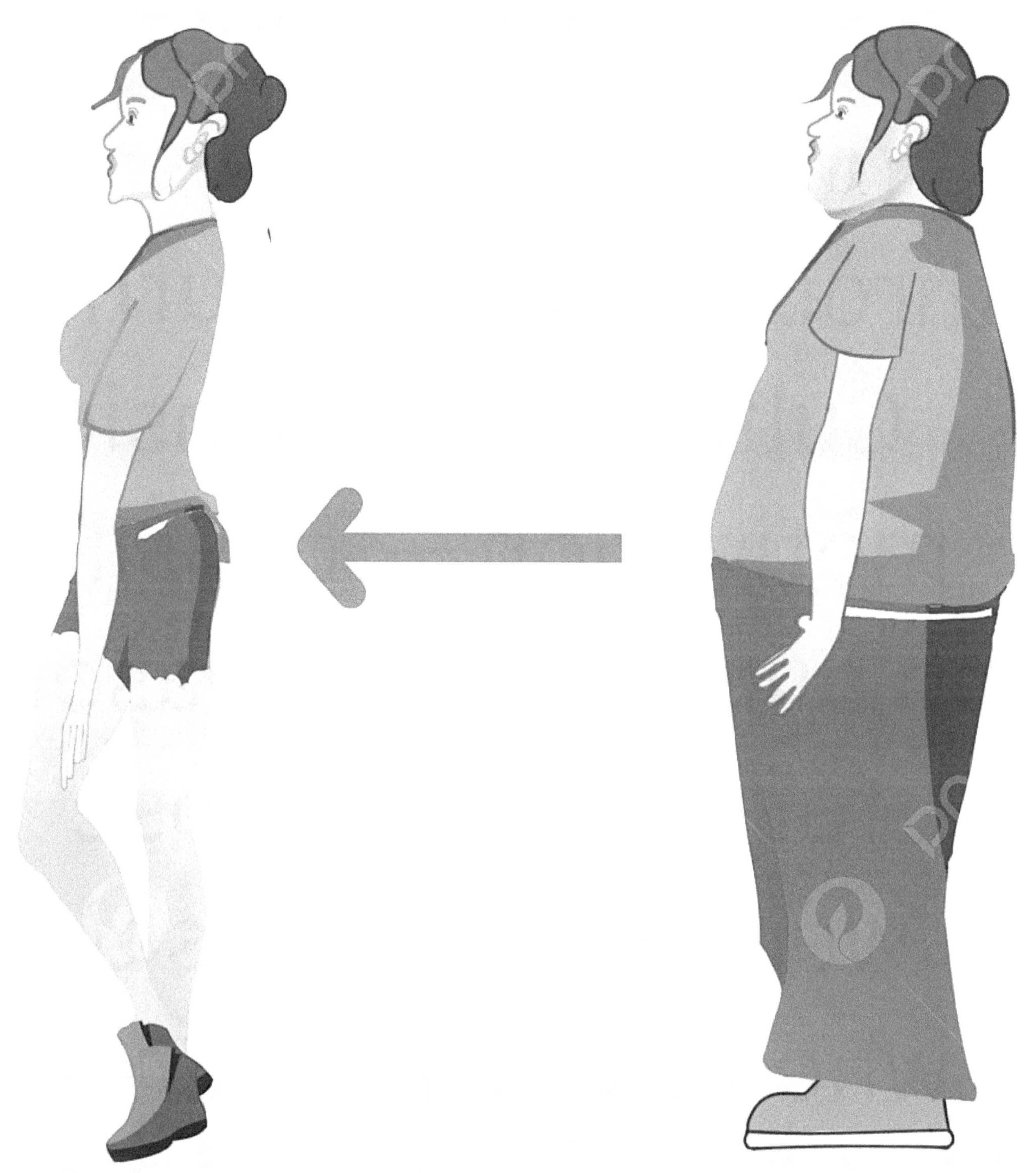

Chapter 21: Finding Motivation

Motivation ebbs and flows throughout our journey. Cultivating intrinsic motivation – focusing on our personal reasons for wanting to lose weight – sustains us when external factors waver

Chapter 22: Celebrating Non-Scale Victories

Non-scale victories, such as increased energy, improved mood, or fitting into smaller clothes, are just as significant as reaching a specific weight goal. Acknowledging and celebrating these achievements reinforces our progress

Chapter 23: Balancing Life and Weight Loss

Balancing weight loss efforts with other aspects of life, such as work, family, and social commitments, is essential for long-term success. Prioritizing self-care and finding a sustainable routine ensure we maintain equilibrium.

Chapter 24: Navigating Social Situations

Social gatherings and events often revolve around food, presenting challenges for those trying to lose weight. Planning ahead, setting boundaries, and focusing on socializing rather than eating help us navigate these situations with confidence

Chapter 25: Staying Positive

Maintaining a positive mindset, even in the face of setbacks, fosters resilience and perseverance. Practicing gratitude, self-compassion, and reframing challenges as opportunities for growth keeps us moving forward

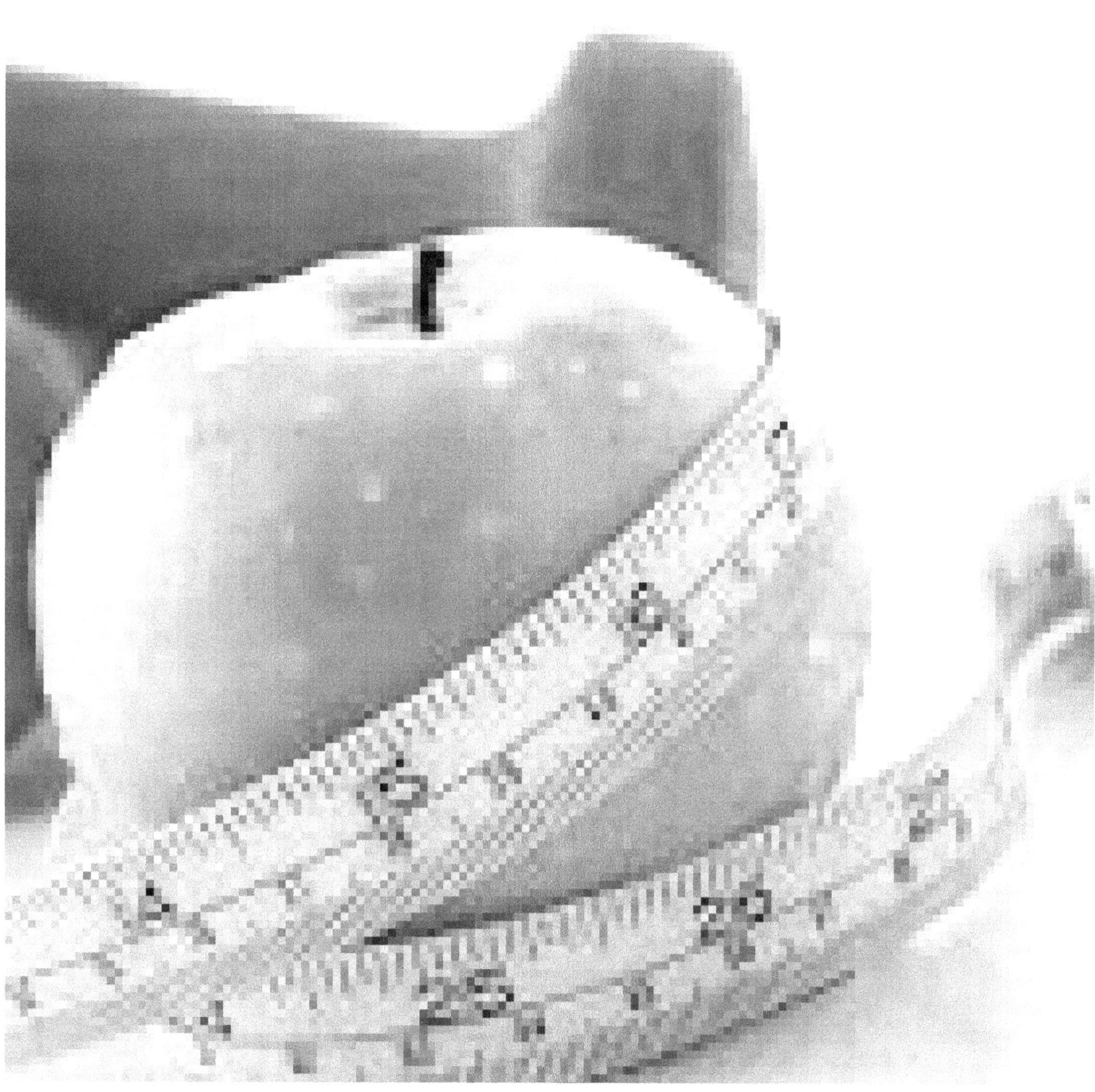

Chapter 26: Cultivating Self-Compassion

Self-compassion is the foundation of self-care and resilience. Treating ourselves with kindness and understanding, especially during difficult times, promotes emotional well-being and fosters a healthy relationship with ourselves.

Chapter 27: Continuing the Journey

Weight loss is not a destination but a lifelong journey. Embracing the process, staying open to growth, and committing to ongoing self-improvement ensure we continue evolving and thriving.

Chapter 28: Conclusion

As we reach the end of this journey, we reflect on how far we've come and look ahead to the possibilities that await. Remember, the journey to weight loss is not always easy, but it's always worth it.

Chapter 29: Exploring Intermittent Fasting

Intermittent fasting has gained popularity for its potential weight loss benefits. By alternating between periods of eating and fasting, we can regulate calorie intake, improve metabolic health, and promote fat loss.

Chapter 30: Incorporating Mindful Movement

Exercise doesn't have to be structured or intense to be effective. Mindful movement practices like yoga, tai chi, or simply taking a daily walk not only burn calories but also reduce stress and enhance overall well-being.

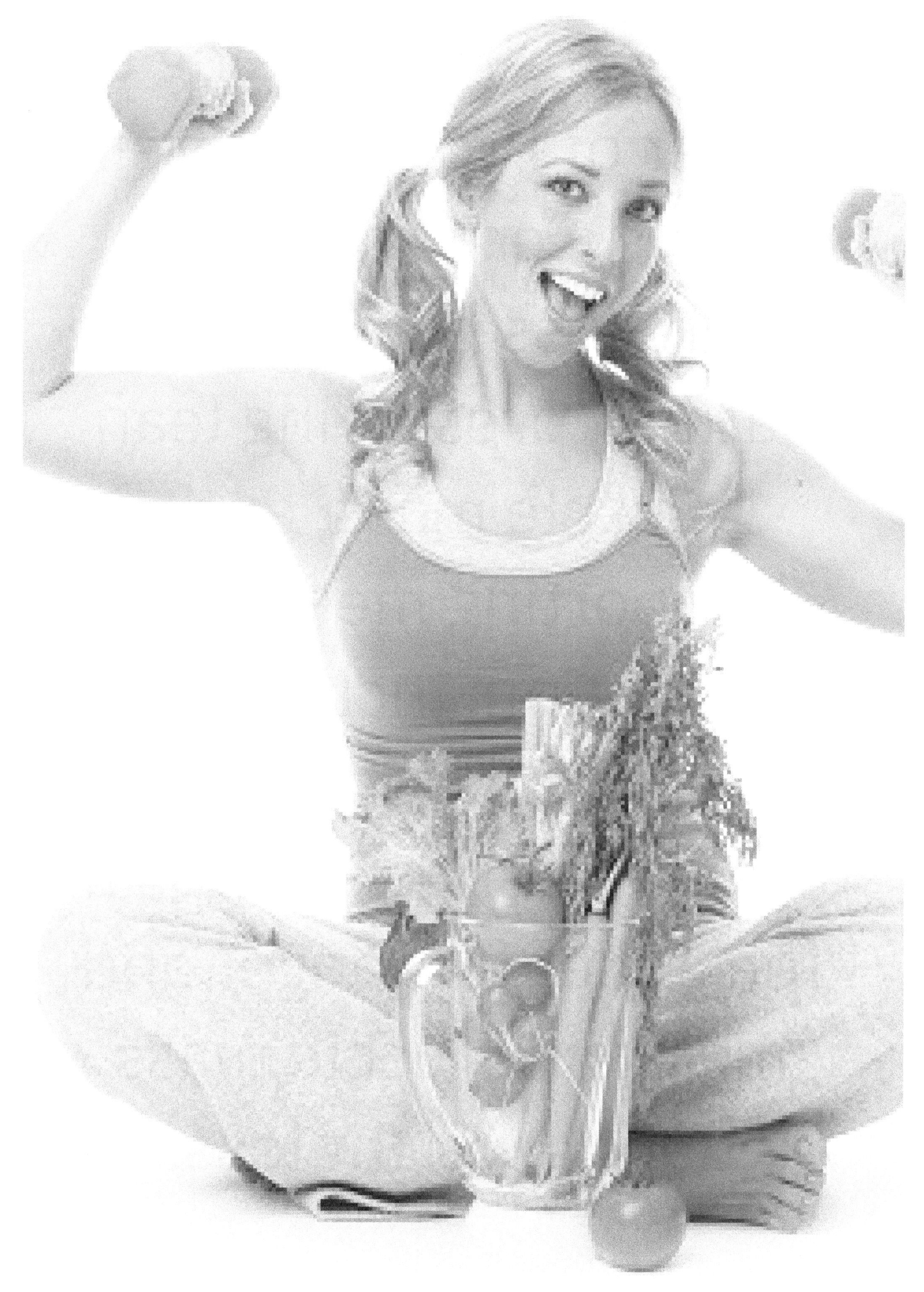

Chapter 31: Harnessing the Power of Protein

Protein plays a crucial role in weight loss by promoting satiety, preserving lean muscle mass, and supporting metabolic function. Including protein-rich foods in our meals and snacks helps us feel fuller for longer and maintain muscle mass during weight loss.

Chapter 32: Exploring Dietary Patterns

Various dietary patterns, such as the Mediterranean diet, plant-based diet, or low-carb diet, offer different approaches to weight loss. Experimenting with different dietary styles allows us to find what works best for our preferences and lifestyle.

Chapter 33: Addressing Emotional Triggers

Emotional triggers can lead to overeating or unhealthy eating habits. By identifying our triggers and developing alternative coping mechanisms, such as journaling, deep breathing, or seeking support from loved ones, we can break free from emotional eating patterns.

Chapter 34: Practicing Portion Control

Portion control is essential for weight loss success. Learning to recognize appropriate portion sizes and practicing mindful eating techniques, such as chewing slowly and savoring each bite, helps us avoid overeating and stay on track with our goals.

Chapter 35: Understanding Metabolism

Metabolism plays a significant role in weight management. Understanding how factors like age, genetics, and lifestyle habits influence metabolism empowers us to make informed choices that support metabolic health and weight loss.

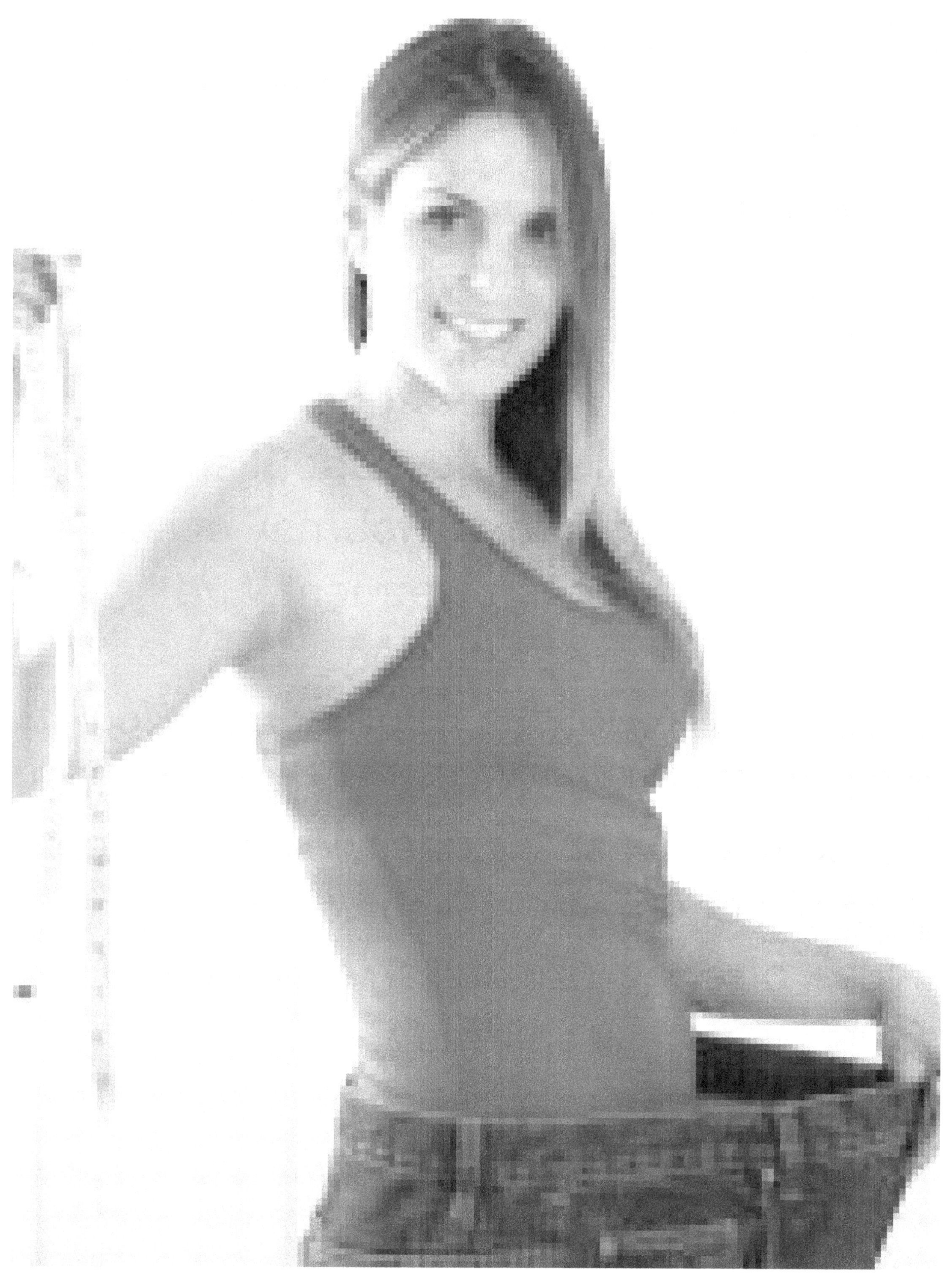

Title: A Holistic Approach to Weight Loss: 82 Chapters of Transformation

In a world inundated with fad diets, quick fixes, and unrealistic expectations, the journey to weight loss can often feel overwhelming and daunting. Yet, at its core, weight loss is not just about shedding pounds; it's a profound journey of self-discovery, empowerment, and transformation.

Welcome to "A Holistic Approach to Weight Loss: 82 Chapters of Transformation." In this comprehensive guide, we delve deep into the multifaceted aspects of weight loss, offering insights, strategies, and inspiration